THE IMPORTANCE OF SUPPLEMENTS AND VITAMINS

What You Need To Know About Supplements

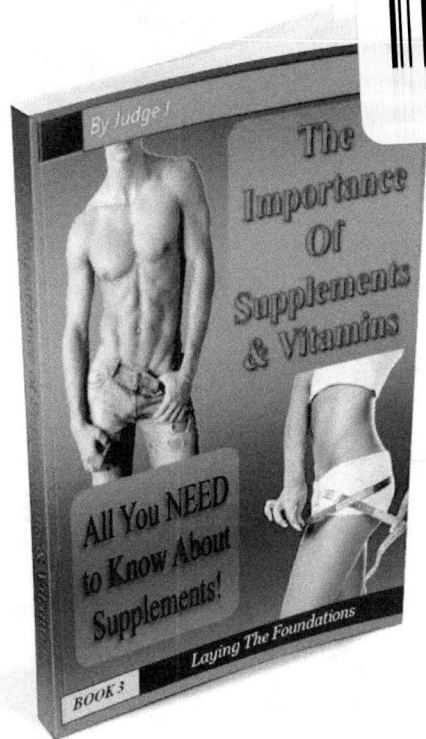

By Judge J

Supplements Can Make ALL The Difference When Trying to Lose Weight or Build Muscle Mass.

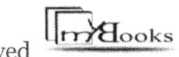

INDEX

Introduction

Supplements are required by our bodies to function at pick performance. They are a mystery to most, and it's this mystery I what to explore with you in this book. So what lead me into the fascinating world of *'Supplements'*?

I have been involved in keeping fit for over 50yrs; it started back in my school days when I fall in love with gymnastics. I went on to study martial arts at the age of 15, and then began bodybuilding in my 20's.

I have spent over 40yrs passing on this experience to others and would like to do the same for you.

This book represents my personal views and experience's, which have been built up over that 50yrs.

I have seen people that have excelled at losing weight and triumphed over their fitness, but I have also seen my fair share of people who despite all their hard work... failed.

Throughout my journey I have found myself asking the following question, *'Why is it that some people succeed when others just cannot make it past the winning post'*.

There are a number of obvious reasons why this is, a lack of willingness to do what needs to be done, to believing that they know better than everyone else, for example.

But there are a number of less obvious reasons why someone may fail too, which should be taken into account before starting any weight loss or fitness routine.

Anything from their age, health, diet, fitness levels, to diabetes.

I discovered from my studies that the two most common factors that interfere with people's ability to succeed in their inability to control, or lose weight, first is the age factor and / or their poor diets.

These two factors started me on a journey to find out what, and if indeed anything could be done to rectify these two problems. Believe it or not, but I found that these two factors actually go hand-in-hand.

Let me explain, the greater your age, the more your body goes through some pretty horrendous changes. It becomes less capable of dealing with the stresses put upon it by dieting, exercise, and every life.

The same can be said for a poor diet too. Your body requires Proteins, vitamins, and minerals to produce energy, help repair and replace damaged cells, and fight off infections.

The less of these compounds you consume, the more your body will become stressed, leading to conditions like fatigue.

The answer to this problem is to take these compounds in the form of Supplementation and vitamins. They are crucial in the fight to manage good health and burn off body fat.

If you train with weights, then it becomes even more crucial to take supplementation and vitamins.

Hard training will deplete your body stores even quicker, and therefore, it's crucial that you replace these elements as quickly as possible, and the only way is through supplementation.

Increased innovations in fitness and weight training, over the past few years, have re-kindled a new resurgence of interest in supplementation and vitamins.

There is no doubt about it, research and a better understanding of supplements have helped those who train their bodies, realize better results a lot quicker!

However, with this new found resurgence comes a problem that most people find hard to overcome when researching supplements... **your need to become a lab nerd**.

The problem is this, it's because almost impossible to keep-up with the latest research and products hitting our shelves on a daily bases.

It's becoming very hard to figure out what the compounds are in these supplements, do they really work, how do you sort out the hype from fact, or, will it be a good fit for your goals...getting fit, or losing that weight.

This is the reason *'why'* I decided to write this book, to give you the full facts, secrets, and insider information, hopefully helping to guide you to a better purchasing decision.

Unfortunately, the supplementation market is full of scams, and companies take advantage of people's ignorance when it comes to understanding what a supplement is.

What does it really do, does it contain the correct quantities and blends of supplements to do the job, is it extracted from the best part of the plant.

These are just a few of the pitfalls in deciding, which supplements to buy.

Hopefully, together we will learn how to guard against the worst practices and embrace the correct elements to help build a good foundation for your weight loss, fitness, and management routine.

Let's start by examining the worst practices you are likely to come across when doing your research.

Starting with 'Fitness Magazines'

The most important thing you should understand about the fitness magazine industry, right off the bat.

The magazine industry realized a long time ago that more money could be made selling supplements than selling advertising space, or, subscriptions in their magazines.

Unfortunately, it doesn't end there, because here's another dirty little *Secret* they don't want you to know about.

It's to do with the fact that most people can't tell where an editorial ends and the advertising begins. It's not your fault, it's the way our brains are wired, and, **'Yes'** you guessed it, it's designed to target this trait.

Look, editorials are more believable than advertising...fact!

Ever noticed how many magazine articles concentrate on the latest, greatest 'breakthroughs' in supplements?

These so called articles aren't really articles at all; they are little more than advertisement masquerading as an article.

They will even throw in 0800 (Free numbers), or, get your free sample, for easy ordering... how convenient is that?

You may be surprised to learn that many people, especially beginners, believe every word they read in these 'Fitness magazines'.

They full for their traps, buying hundreds, thousands of dollars worth of useless supplements, or 'Fat burning pills', powders, and drinks, as a result.

Magazines are there to make a profit, and form their advertising revenues it's clear that there is much profit to be made from promoting supplements like crazy.

It doesn't matter to the fitness magazines, whether or not a supplement works, as long as the supplement company keeps on advertising in their pages.

And here's a dirty little **Secret** that these magazines are desperate to keep under wraps, most of these fitness magazines actually <u>OWN</u> the supplement companies they advertise in their pages.... talk about making a killing.

This is why you see so many supplement advertisements in these magazines, the more they advertise, the more the supplements sell, and on and on the cycle goes.

It's not about presenting you with the best supplements, it's all about... Profits!

How to recognize a good quality 'Supplement'

You can train for years and never see cuts in your abs. You can spend thousands of pounds on supplements that claim to burn fat and increase your energy levels.

You have seen people in the gym who've tried hard and spent their hard earned money in the hope of producing those wash board like abs...

Who end-up becoming very dejected and disillusioned with their results and their training altogether?

For this reason I have made it one of my life's quests to find out more about these supplements, and the supplement companies who make such extravagant claims regarding their products.

Why? Because I was once one of those people who lost pounds from my pockets and not from my waist line.

I'm not saying that there aren't some good reputable companies out there, there are, but they are far and few between.

How do you recognize a good quality supplement, compared to ingredients whose affects our very questionable?

It goes without saying, today there are hundreds, if not thousands of different supplements on the market, all claiming to be the best of the best, how do you decide, which supplements are right for you?

In this book I will be concentrating on the facts behind fat-burning, energy, and the most controversial supplement claim of all... testosterone boosting supplements.

Let's take a hypothetical look at a blend of fat-burning supplements.

In this example, the product contains 5mcg of Ephedra, 200mcg of caffeine, 20mcg of L-Carnitine, and 25mcg of Chromium Picolinate, this is the typical average dosage you'll find on the market today.

At first glance this blend may look-up to the job of burning body fat, but is it?

You definitely would get a big blast of caffeine, but unfortunately, the reality is the other ingredients don't add up too much and won't do much for you either...the dosage is just way too low.

Let's say you paid £20 for the product, what you're really paying for is **£20** for a **<u>Caffeine</u>** shot or a cup of coffee!

It's very difficult for the average consumer to recognize a product of high quality, which has been well-designed, simply, because very few of us are trained chemists.

It's very easy for companies to confuse and misdirect people when it comes to using scientific terminology and mumbo-jumbo... how would you know the difference between a scientific fact, or their sales pitch.

The fact is most supplement companies will figure out their profit margins first, by calculating the cost of the production, packaging, and distribution costs... and <u>then</u> manufacture the product accordingly.

On the other hand, a good supplement company will put together blends that are based upon some sort of actual scientific research, and then decide the cost to the customer.

As you can appreciate this will increase the cost of the supplement, but in this case quality is far better than quantity.

So 'What' should you be on the lookout for

When looking at any of the products labels on the market today, it's very difficult to know just what it is you're looking at.

Well here lies the dilemma and supplements companies know this only too well.

You see these supplement companies know and rely on the fact that you have no idea how effective, safe, or whether its top grade quality.

Unfortunately, most supplements are just not that effective, or simply don't measure up to the claims they make on their bottle, but it gets worse than that, because some don't do any of what the label claims!

So what can you do to make sure you don't end-up spending your hard earned money on products that will leave you disappointed?

Your first step is to examine closely what's is exactly 'Written' on the label

For example, have you any idea what the difference is between what is called the whole herb and the '**Herbal extract**'?

'**Herbal extract**' relates to the part of the plant, which contains the active ingredient you're looking at.

The rest of the plant, **98%**, will have no active ingredient within it and will have no effect on your body at all.

That's, because 'herbal extracts' costs a great deal more than using the whole plant...companies who put profit first will always opt to use the whole plant to keep their costs down.

So it's important that you concentrate on looking for supplements that contain a high percentage of the 'herbal extract' and not the rest of the plant.

The second thing you should be looking at is the supplements 'Dosage'

'Why', because the higher the percentage of *'herbal extract'* there is in the supplements, the more it will dramatically **decrease** the number of capsules that is required for your daily intake.

And the strength and concentration of the active ingredients can be increased by up to **20** times the power of the original herb.

Or you could simply waste your money by opting for extracts that involve the whole plant in its production (they are usually much cheaper) by **not** taking enough.

Tip: Rule of thumb

All supplement companies print the daily intake (dosage recommendations) on their labels, so note the dosage.

If the dosage recommended is **three** or **four** capsules a day then that's a pretty good indication that you will be throwing your money away.

The third thing you need to examine is its 'Elemental Values'

This value will be the amount of actual ingredient there is in each tablet. If we take *'Chromium Picolinate'*, for example, then on the label you may read 200 mg of calcium picolinate per tablet.

This could very well-mean that you are only getting 24 mg of the mineral chromium (12% (value) of 200mg).

The minimum amount you require is **400** mg to be effective, but as you can see from our example you are only getting 24 mg of this ingredient... it's not going to work!

At this level you would have to consume around 18 capsules a day just to get the right amount to do any good.

It's important to know that this value holds true for all supplements, so if you base your decisions on cost then you may very well be doing yourself out of money, and stripping away any benefits you hoped to gain.

What else should I be mindful of

All pharmaceutical drugs will put a strain on various parts of your body, and upping your dosage believing it would work better, will increase any of the supplements side-effects.

Unfortunately, because of the high costs involved, most supplement companies omit to include all of the required information, or, additional ingredients to combat their affects.

For example, a well designed fat-burning supplement should contain extra ingredients to support the '**Adrenal Glands**' and the '**Thyroid**'.

Unfortunately, these ingredients are very expensive and most supplement companies will opt to leave them out.

Supplements that contain supportive ingredients are always going to cost you more, but with them the effects will be far more powerful and well worth the price.

If you are going to take a fat-burning supplement, for example, then you need to know and understand that supplements will make your body extract or use up minerals, like magnesium, at a far greater rate and therefore, should be included within the supplement.

It's also important they contain nutrients that will support, or increase '**Fatty Acid**' usage too.

Also where possible, and if its within your budget range, the supplement should contain nutrients that will help fight off '**free radicals**', as those cell destroyers will increase due to an increase metabolism rate from your exercise.

And last, but not least, wherever possible, you should aim to buy supplements that support nutrients that will help to regulate blood sugar and insulin levels, **'Why'**, because insulin levels are essential to fat loss.

Although many of these extra minerals will not be found in your choice of fat-burning supplements, you should however, consider taking these nutrients separately.

Incidentally, if you are looking for a fat-burning supplement, make sure to take '**Chromium Polynicotinate**' and '**Vanady Sulphate**', as both of these nutrients will help the fatty acids to cross the cell walls into the mitochondria, to be used as energy, it will not be stored as fat.

Many people take '**Chromium**' on a daily basis, but because **chromium** can enhance insulin sensitivity and affect glucose levels, diabetics and hypoglycamics, should consult their doctors before taking a course.

'**L-Carnitine**' is also an essential mineral, as is '**Magnesium**', '**Copper**' and '**Potassium**', for thyroid and adrenal support.

As I have already mentioned, consuming more minerals raises the metabolism rate, this increased activity creates more '**free radicals**', consequently it makes it very important to include a good anti-oxidant agent into your daily diet. One such agent is '**Calcium D-Glucarate**', and another is '**Milk Thistle**', or '**Hawthorn berry**'.

You should also consider '**Green Tea**' as it contains **40%** 'Polyphenols' (the most abundant antioxidants), which is a very powerful anti-oxidant and anti-cancer agent... they block the action of enzymes that cancers need for growth.

A multipurpose vitamin and mineral tablet should be included too, because as mentioned before, these fat-burning supplements extracts, will force your system to burn them at a much higher rate.

You should also consider adding aspirin to your fat burning ingredients, because it's been demonstrated to categorically increase the fat burning potential of the Ephedra (a plant, which is valued as an herbal remedy by the Chinese) and caffeine mix.

Alternatively, you could use *'Salix alba'*, which is closely related chemically and pharmacologically, to aspirin, and can be used in addition to aspirin or as a standalone.

Increasing Supplement levels takes time

It doesn't matter whether you are building muscle, fat burning, energy development, power lifting, or keeping fit, taking supplements covers a pretty hefty field, and yet there are several factors that go into optimizing your growth...

It is important to remember that all supplements take '**TIME**' for it to reach the optimum levels, within the body, to have any affect what's-so-ever.

Don't expect to see results within a few weeks.

There is however, a specific supplement that will support and enhance whatever activity you are into. Above we targeted fat-burners; below we will take a look at some of the best supplements around today.

For example, as you know muscle is increased through a combination of training to the max, stimulating various muscle fibres, increasing anabolic hormones, avoiding muscle loss, getting a pump, etc.

So it's pretty obvious that you need to tap into the most powerful muscle growth potential possible, and it's a sure bet for those who are serious about their results, they take the best combination stack possible to work synergistically, and help you reach your goals faster.

PROVEN: List of Body Enhancing Supplements to Include in Your Daily Dietary Requirements...

Although, I can't list ALL the possible supplements that are available to you in this book, there are far too many, I will discuss the ones I feel are the most important for you to consider.

There are around 10 known, approved, and trusted Growth Factors and fat-burning supplements that have stood the test of time.

There have been numerous studies to back-up the results and demonstrate by those who have taken them. A word of warning, it's been my experience, and that of others, that most of the new, next supplement breakthroughs tend to be more hype that action.

Supplements help aid your program for fat burning, muscle exploding, rip roaring, cardiovascular endurance, which complement each other and will make the perfect stack.

Remember to always read the labels, warnings, and directions, provided with the product before using or consuming the product...

CREATINE

Get Stronger by Taking 'Creatine'

'Creatine' is a supplement that's been studied more than any other supplement around today. It is a natural nitrogenous organic acid we all have stored in our muscles, but there isn't enough to create any growth after training.

To get stronger, you need to work hard and lift heavy weights...period, but that puts a huge strain on your body, and sometimes we need help to push on.

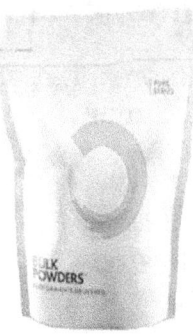

'Creatine' as been around for some time now, and is one of the only supplements to have proven its worth, over and over, again. Supplements containing Creatine offer you your best chance to increase your power during your workouts, increasing the number of plates you lift.

This increase in lifting capacity will allow you to hit your **Type II** muscle fibres harder, triggering much faster strength gains.

However, words of warning...

Stay away from the fancy named Creatine... Ethyl-Esther, a version that's been promoted heavily.

'Why' because...**it's a total scam!**

Remember to stick with good plain old Creatine-monohydrate, or if you're really adventurous, Creatine-gluconate.

If you take Creatine in a powder form, which I recommend, it gets absorbed into your system much quicker.

Also remember to take it as soon as you mix it up, because it starts to disintegrate as soon as it comes into contact with water.

Creatine takes time to build up in your body, it may take a couple of weeks before you show your maximum gains in strength and performance.

Creatine is water soluble and will therefore; clear the system in a short period of time. Whatever you do, don't stop taking creatine, not even on none training days.

Creatine is safe and can be taken for as long as you wish, but it is advisable to take a break from taking it from time to time...

Tips:

** When I break from taking Creatine, I do this when I'm about to cycle to lighter weights and higher reps, about every 4 weeks, for 2 weeks, when I cycle back to heavy compound weights again.

** Also, avoid exceeding the recommended dosage when loading-up, as this will result in many involuntary urgent visits to the toilet.

Creating Monohydrate is the world's most tested, number one muscle bulking and strength building supplement on the market today...

I'm asked everyday to recommend a supplement to my reader's.

And although I don't like to do this, because I don't want to earn money from selling supplements, I will however, do some of the heavy lifting for you.

I have no connection with, or manufacture, any of these supplements. I will however, give you my best recommended 'Buys', and a link at the end of each review to the best supplement that meets all the above criteria's.

To read more information about this supplement, please copy this link into your browser...

http://increasemusclesize.net/creatine

L-ARGININE

Build Massive Muscle Mass & Burn Fat

'L-Arginine' is the best supplement for creating a pump, **'Yes'**, do you remember why you need to get a pump when you work out?

Well it's, because the pump helps to contribute to muscle growth by flooding the muscle with oxygen and nutrient rich blood essential to muscle repair.

L-Arginine is a vasodilator that helps to increase the blood flow in the body, allowing you to achieve a BETTER pump, and importantly maintain it for longer period during your training... just what the bodybuilder ordered.

The pump feels great, looks good and ... **builds muscle**!

L-Arginine is a commonly occurring amino acid, which is found naturally in the human body and carries out a large number of essential positive jobs throughout the body.

L-Arginine is an Amino acid, they are the building blocks that links together to form proteins, and as we all know, muscles require proteins to grow.

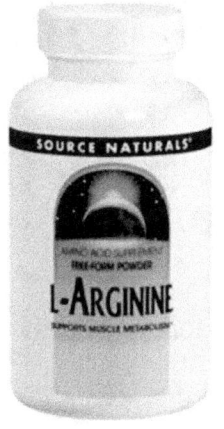

The body also uses Arginine to produce nitric oxide (NO), very important to a bodybuilder. How does Arginine work? Well put in a nut shell, it helps the blood vessels to relax, and indeed several other effects in the body. The vasodilator effect of Arginine is one of the most important factors to consider, because it helps to maintain a healthy blood flow around the body.

This is important as the blood carries oxygen and nutrients to the muscles during training, helping to start muscle recovery during your session and maintaining good cardiovascular performance.

For the first time trainer, it's useful, because of the extra blood flow, getting more oxygen to their muscles lowering the onset of fatigue.

Also the reduction in estrogen lowering their fat levels will also help to achieve quicker fitness levels.

It's also been known now for many years that Arginine speeds up the healing process of wounds and muscle damage.

As we all know any form of aggressive exercise will breakdown muscle fibres, and for bodybuilders this process is essential for muscle growth.

There are studies still being carried out today on the possible performance benefits of L-Arginine.

The great news is that results are still being echoed on what's already known about this incredible supplement. Research is ongoing into the other possible benefits of taking this supplement, but so far it's looking equally promising.

When taken post-workout, this supplement has been shown to increase a person's ability, increase their performance for short, high impact exercise, increasing the intensity and duration.

This has also been demonstrated to be especially beneficial in those between the ages of 30 to 50.

Arginine has also shown many positive results when used as part of a weight loss regime, helping people to drop their body fat levels.

Research has established that Arginine acquires energy for muscle growth, rather than fat storage.

L-Arginine has also demonstrated its ability to increase sexual arousal.

Arginine is without doubt an exceptional supplement for helping to improve your performance, and overall health, and should be included into your list of supplements to take.

L-Arginine is a must for muscle growth; we recommend the following brand, because it ticks all the right boxes and has been on trial with us.

To read more information about this supplement, please copy this link into your browser...

http://increasemusclesize.net/l-arginine

CALCIUM D-GLUCARATE

Best Way to Rid Your Body of Harmful Toxins

It's been shown in studies to defend cellular health in all of the major organs.

Aids the body in the abstraction of many harmful toxins, and helps to lower abnormally high levels of steroid hormones including estrogen, testosterone, and progesterone.

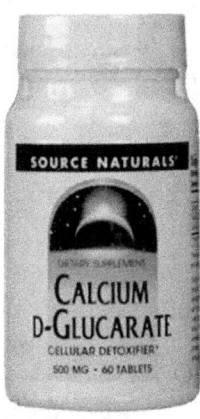

Calcium D-Glucarate is especially useful for lowering the estrogen build-up in men. Estrogen dominance causes weight gain around the belly, butt, thighs, chest, and hips. This can have a devastating effect on the male physiologically, trapping and retaining water, increasing Gynecomastia (male boobs).

This is a common condition that causes boys and men's breasts to swell and become larger than normal.

Estrogen robs men of achieving their weight loss goals to get ripped or look healthier.

This is because estrogen piles on the fat and water, giving your body that puffed or bloated look.

Also, in woman progesterone levels begin to rapidly decline, increasing their hormone level imbalance leading to the same bloating and weight gain effect.

So it's essential to get rid of this build-up of estrogen in the early stages of dieting, and Calcium D-Glucarate will help support normal hormonal levels.

There have been many studies and a lot of research, which has also shown that Calcium D-glucarate shows promise as an anti-cancer agent. When taking Calcium D-Glucarate you should increase your calcium levels.

For example include: dark green leafy vegetables, dairy products, and calcium-fortified cereals, apples, broccoli, brussel sprouts, cabbage, kale, and oranges.

If you are having problems moving weight, or feeling blotted, then you may be suffering from a build-up of toxins, or a Hormonal imbalance.

Get your supply of Calcium D-Glucarate, please copy this link into your browser...

http://increasemusclesize.net/calcium-d-glucarate

L-GLUTAMINE

Increase HGH Levels - STOP Muscle Breakdown

'L-Glutamine' is the most abundant amino acid to be found in your muscles. L-Glutamine can be found in **61%** of skeletal muscle of, which **19%** is nitrogen, making it the primary transporter of nitrogen into your muscle cells.

Not only does L-Glutamine transform nitrogen into your muscles, but it plays a crucial role in protein synthesis, cell volumizing, and anti-catabolism.

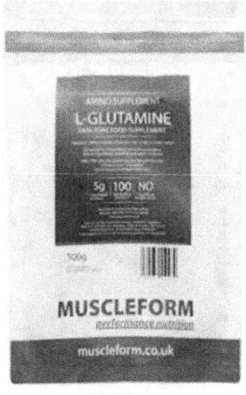

This anti catabolism effect is very important as this STOPS you losing muscle mass.

Remember that I mentioned that muscles act like little furnaces, helping to burn off body fat. So hanging on to as much muscle as possible, is crucial in the fight to burn off your body fat.

The problem is that during heavy intense weight training, L-Glutamine levels are greatly depleted, which diminishes your strength, stamina and recovery times. It can take up to 6 days for levels to return to normal.

Studies and research has shown that L-Glutamine supplementation can help to reduce muscle breakdown, and improve protein metabolism.

This is a particularly useful tool in the fight to reduce body fat levels without losing any muscle...

There is nothing worse than jumping on the scales only to realize that your weight loss is in muscle and not fat.

Taking L-Glutamine can increase growth hormone levels by **400%**.

L-Glutamine is also needed throughout your body for optimal performance.

Especially the transportation of ammonia to the liver, where it is converted into less toxic urea and then excreted by the kidneys.

Ammonia is a toxic metabolic by-product of protein breakdown, which obstructs the muscle repair process.

Don't let muscle catabolism rob you of all your hard work.

For more information, or to grab your supply, please copy this link into your browser... http://mybooksupply.com/wp/l-glutamine

BACC

One of The Most Important Amino Acids To Take

BCAA' (Branched Chain Amino Acids) are the basic building blocks of protein, which are of special importance to bodybuilders, power athletes, and those trying to lose weight.

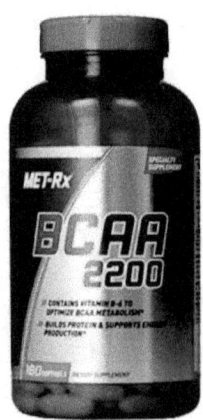

Everyone who is trying to lose excess fat are fully aware of the excellent benefits of following a high protein program, low carbs diet. Around **33%** of muscle protein consists of **BCAAs**, and most diets don't always contain enough protein to do the job of repairing the fibres broken down during exercise.

Also most people don't understand that even when they are doing a moderate amount of exercise this can cause levels of BCAAs to drop rapidly, resulting in muscle tissue breakdown or catabolism, and fatigued.

There are many benefits associated with taking BACC's, just to name a few:

** Studies have shown that people consuming BCAA's with all meals have less visceral belly fat and much more muscle mass.
** BCAAs promotes protein synthesis and inhibits the breakdown of muscle cells.
** BCAAs also help's to improve glucose uptake and insulin sensitivity, improving the metabolic rate.
** Research as shown that taking BCAAs before exercise, dramatically improves muscle and energy production.
** BCAAs dramatically reduces muscle soreness after exercise.
** BCAAs also dramatically improves recovery time when fatigued.

Research has shown that taking BCAA's had a dramatic effect on the levels of anabolic hormones like testosterone, insulin, and growth hormone (HGH).

This is important, because these hormones are responsible for the repair and the growth of muscle cells.

Taking BCAA's post training helps to keep the levels of all these anabolic hormones high.

Anabolic hormones are normally elevated during exercise, but crash, way below the baseline after training.

This dramatically decreases their ability to affect repairs and recovery after training?

Also, the studies have clearly shown this affect to remain elevated for several hours after training.

Some new research has shown, when on a fat loss diet, taking BCAA's seemed to maximize fat loss, it would seem

BCAAs have the ability to spare glycogen and increase insulin sensitivity, speeding up the results of a fat loss plan.

BACC's aids muscle growth, strengthen, and has a sufficient impact on muscle recovery.

Taking BCAA supplementation is therefore, very beneficial and important for bodybuilders, power athletes, and those trying to lose weight, to take as part of their supplementation program.

For more information or purchase your own supply, please copy this link into your browser...

http://mybooksupply.com/wp/bcaa

FLAX SEED OIL

Not all Fats Are Bad For You – The Seeds of Life

'Flax Seed Oil', unrefined. Flax Seed Oil is rich in the Omega 3 essential fatty acid (EFA), alpha-linolenic acid typically **50-65%**.

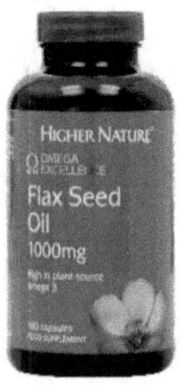

It is also a good source of Omega 6 and Omega 9, and contains mixed tocopherols (especially gamma tocopherol) and tocotrienols.
Omega 3 and 6 supports a healthy heart, arteries and brain.
Fatty acids make up the walls of every cell in the body and make hormone-like substances, important for many essential body processes.

Benefits to taking Flax Seed Oil...

** Lowers High cholesterol

** Helps prevent heart disease

** Can help improve dry eye in people   with Sjogren's syndrome

** Plays a vital role in burning body fat

** Increases Athletic performance and recovery after training.

Flaxseed oil aids in the optimization of all metabolic and physiologic processes in your body, and using flax seed oil on a regular basis helps you lose weight naturally.

It's important to make sure that your supply of flax seed oil is produced by a process known as cold-pressed.

Most manufacturers use heat to extract the oils from the flax seeds, along with their nutrients, to use in their products.

This process of using heat to extract the oils destroys many of the good, beneficial, components in the plant.

You need to make sure that the flax seed oil you're going to use as been extracted using the process of cold-pressed.

You will pay a little bit more for this method of extracting the oils, but its well worth the cost.

If you are looking to take Flax Seed Oil as part of your dietary supplementation, please copy this link into your browser...

http://mybooksupply.com/wp/fax-seed-oil

CHROMIUM

More Important Than You Might Think

'Chromium' is a mineral supplement that helps to promote Fat, Protein & Sugar metabolism. Chromium helps to turn fats, carbohydrates, and proteins into energy.

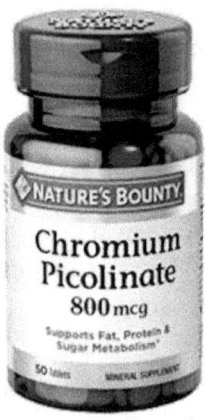

Therefore, it is important to introduce some exercise into your daily routine if you are looking to gain benefits from this supplement. There is some research that has shown Chromium may increase 'good' HDL cholesterol. There are also studies that indicate that Chromium may be very instrumental in building muscle, burning fat, and helping the body to use its stored carbohydrates.

Chromium is known to enhance the action of insulin, helping to maintain a higher metabolism rate, and actively helping to correct glucose intolerance and insulin resistance.

Optimal glucose and insulin functions are required to aid burning fat and building muscle mass.

However, you should not take Chromium on its own to reduce or increase fat burning or muscle mass, it should be taken with other supplements in order to enhance its effects.

In terms of safety more data is needed, but you should try to source it from a well balanced diet.

You can get your daily supply from food sources such as coffee, oysters, cereals, potatoes, peas, rye, whole grains, beer, brewer's yeast, tea, thyme, and processed meats.

Remember that training will lower your mineral levels and therefore, there is some justification for taking Chromium, short term, to boost levels.

For more information or to purchase your own supply, please copy this link into your browser...

http://mybooksupply.com/wp/chromium

RHODIOLA ROSEA

The Holy Grail For Losing Weight

'Rhodiola-rosea', first came to my attention through a study looking into the possible effect it might have had on increasing memory and learning.

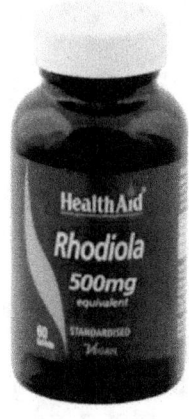

I then read another report showing how effective it was at increasing energy and decreasing mental fatigue.
But the paragraph that grabbed my attention the most was the one that explained how Rhodiola dealt with fat cells. This really got my attention.
You may or may not know, but body fat is stored in the adipose tissue. When fat gets stored in this tissue, it becomes very hard to get rid of.

That's why some people just can't seem to get rid of certain fatty spots, including 'love handles' or a fatty 'tyre' around the abdomen.

The body contains an enzyme called hormone-sensitive lipase, which is able to break down fat stored in adipose tissue.

The body contains an enzyme called hormone-sensitive lipase, which is able to break down fat stored in adipose tissue.

But this enzyme is not especially active, and this is where Rhodiola rosea comes in.

Extracts of Rhodiola rosea have the capacity to activate hormone-sensitive lipase, thus increasing the breakdown of fat stored in adipose tissue.

Rosavin specifically contributes to fat breakdown by activating hormone-sensitive lipase, thus increasing the breakdown of fat stored in adipose tissue.

The benefits of taking Rhodiola rosea:

** Can help the body to recover from fatigue and other symptoms associated with chronic stress, or adrenal exhaustion
** Can help to improve cardiovascular health and regulate the heart beat?
** Is antioxidant-rich and helps to rid the body of toxins
** It's also been used to treat trauma, exposure to toxins, fatigue and sleep deprivation, infection, or psychological stress, and has a normalizing, or, balancing effect on the body.

Research has also shown that Rhodiola can reduce the levels of cortisol created during training, and blood sugar aspect of the belly fat equation, because it utilizes the fat stored in abdominal cells.

The fatter and larger the cell becomes, and the bigger and heavier you will weigh...remember you can't reduce the number of cells that are created overtime, only reduce their size.

Cortisol is a killer of muscle mass, because it's the job of cortisol to cannibalize damaged or dead cells ready to be replaced.

And what do we all do when we train...'**Yes'** breakdown muscle fibres.

It doesn't take rocket science to work out that cortisol destroys the very muscle fibres we want to repair.

And the whole reason we break them down in the first place is to have them repair stronger and thicker each time we train for maximum muscle size.

Even if you are just training to reduce fat levels, you don't want to flood your body with cortisol, because you don't want weight loss to be muscle loss, but fat loss.

Cortisol is also known as the 'stress' hormone' the more cortisol, the more stress you are putting your body under. The more the body becomes stressed out the more fat you will deposit into the fat cell.

As with many herbs that increase energy, too high a dosage of Rhodiola rosea can cause side effects.

Rhodiola side effects may include restlessness, irritability, and insomnia, if you find yourself suffering these effects after starting a course... Stop immediately.

For more information or to purchase your own supply, please copy this link into your browser...

http://mybooksupply.com/wp/rhodiola

SIDA CORDIFOLIA

The Strongest Fat Burner, Anti-inflammation, and Antioxidant Around Today

'Sida-cordifolia' is the strongest natural fat loss supplement available today. It's used for the treatment of inflammation, asthma, bronchitis, and nasal congestion.

Sida-cordifolia helps to increase the metabolism rate, raising the core temperature, known as 'Thermogenics' to help burn off calories, increasing your energy and motivation for exercise.

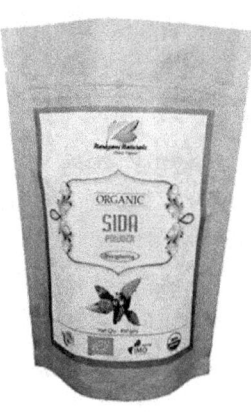

Sida-cordifolia contains small quantities of both ephedrine and pseudoephedrine. The interesting component is the Ephedrine, because it stimulates the central nervous system and this will have an effect on weight loss. Sida-cordifolia may possibly assist in weight loss through its hypoglycaemic activity (blood sugar lowering), reducing the storage of fat within fat cells.

Sida-cordifolia possesses potent antioxidant activity, which as the potential to significantly increase endogenous antioxidants.

Sida-cordifolia has also been shown to possess potent anti-inflammatory activity, which reduces toxin build-up due to inflammation.

It's been discovered that food can have a devastating effect on triggering inflammation, the biggest offenders being processed and sugary foods, as well as Trans-fats, which are present in a variety of snack foods, fried foods, and baked foods.

Inflammation is a natural response to threats from injury, germs, environmental pollutants, stress toxins, and other destructive influences.

Inflammation can be very destructive to our normal cells, irritating and wearing down cartilage and tissues.

Inflammation can also slow down the healing of damaged tissue, preventing their repair, coursing prolonged swelling and pain.

Sida-cordifolia has also demonstrated anti-stress, 'Adaptogenic', and cortisol (The stress hormone) lowering properties too.

Any of which, can prevent and promote further complications.

For more information or to purchase your own supply, please copy this link into your browser...

http://mybooksupply.com/wp/sidacordifolia

FENUGREEK

Maintain Healthy Metabolism, Burn Fat, And Lower Cholesterol

'Fenugreek' is an herb that is commonly found growing in the Mediterranean region.

It's known for its ability to help to maintain a healthy metabolism, increase libido, helps lower blood glucose (sugar) levels, lowers cholesterol, and has many other cardiovascular benefits.

As mentioned before, hormonal imbalance may be a very important factor to consider when you are looking to lose weight, or burn off body fat.

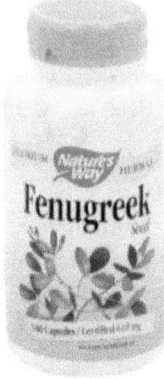

Fenugreek is also used to treat hormonal disorders. Sugar is another very dominant factor in your diet, which as a huge effect upon your body fat levels, and research as shown Fenugreek to be an excellent treatment for significantly lowering blood sugar levels.

As you get older, insulin resistance can start to affect the body's ability to get rid of excessive amounts of sugar circulating in the blood.

Insulin's primary job is to mop up those sugars after eating a meal, and then deliver that sugar to the muscles to be burnt off as fuel when exercising.

But the cells in the muscles start to resist and won't allow the insulin to deliver its glucose load.

The insulin can't retain the glucose and will therefore, must deliver it to the only other cell in the body that will accept the glucose, and that's the fat cell.

This is of course disaster for both the bodybuilder and anyone trying to lose weight.

Fenugreek is well known for its ability to lower sugar levels and should be taken if you suspect you are suffering from insulin resistance.

Fenugreek contains a lot of mucilage, which helps sooth

gastrointestinal inflammation by coating the lining of the stomach and intestine... it's therefore, an effective remedy against heartburn or Acid Reflux.

Fenugreek is a good source of protein, minerals like copper vitamin C, potassium, calcium, iron, selenium, zinc, manganese, magnesium, and Diosgenin.

Poultices and other external formulations have been used for wounds and skin irritations.

For more information or to purchase your own supply, please copy this link into your browser...

http://mybooksupply.com/wp/fenugreek

L-CITRULLINE

A Modern Alternative to 'L-arginine'

The main role of 'L-Citrulline' is to reduce fatigue. It does this by reducing the negative effects of ammonia, which is created during training.

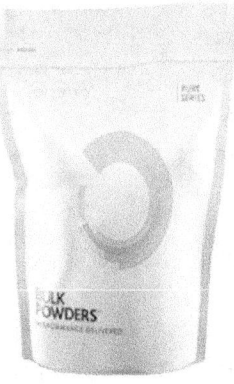

During training any athlete will be looking to optimise blood flow to the tissues, this is important in order to maximize the performance and after training to aid in recovery. And this is where L-Citrulline comes in to its own. It works, because the body is able to convert L-Citrulline to L-Arginine, and then, and this is the important part, it gets converted into nitric-oxide.

This is important, because this conversion to nitric-oxide increases the amount of blood and oxygen they get delivered to the working muscles, preventing physical fatigue.

Also, when you eat protein, the body breaks it down into amino acids; ammonia is produced from leftover amino acids, which must be removed from the body.

This is known as the urea cycle, and L-Citrulline helps to play a major role in this process.

L-Citrulline also aids to reduce the amount of lactic acid build-up you experience in your muscles during your workouts.

A build-up of lactic acid during training, not only slows down your progress, and is painful, but this lactic acid build-up can also have a debilitating effect on the muscles the following day, leading to stiffness and probably a missed training session.

It's important to avoid this lactic acid build-up as it can lead to a build-up of ammonia levels in the body, high levels can stress the kidney, which can become fatal.

Nitric-oxide or **NO**, as it is commonly known, plays a major role in the vascular relaxation (blood pressure, directional dysfunction) immune response, inflammation, response, and memory formation.

What are the benefits of taking L-Citrulline...

- Augments nitric oxide production
- Improves energy and performance
- Reduces muscle soreness after exercise
- Ideal for pre-workout
- Improves performance

Sources of L-Citrulline include watermelons, muskmelons, bitter melons, squashes, gourds, cucumbers, and pumpkins.

For more information or to purchase your own supply, please copy this link into your browser...

http://mybooksupply.com/wp/citrulline

L-HISTIDINE

An Other One You Could Add to Your Arson

'L-Histidine' is a semi-essential amino acid, and has several influences on metabolic reactions in the body.

L-Histidine is involved in the synthesis of haemoglobin, tissue repair and the strengthening of the immune system.

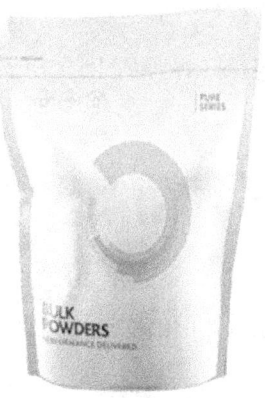

L-Histidine is a powerful blood vessel dilator, which allows more blood and oxygen to flow into your muscles during exercise. The great thing about L-Histidine is its really good at repairing tissue for anyone who trains, regardless of your level, or the exercises you are doing.

We all need to be able to repair the damage we do during training.

For more information or to purchase your own supply, please copy this link into your browser...

GREEN TEA

The Fat Burner and More

Green tea is without doubt one of the healthiest drinks you can consume that's packed full of fantastic goodies.

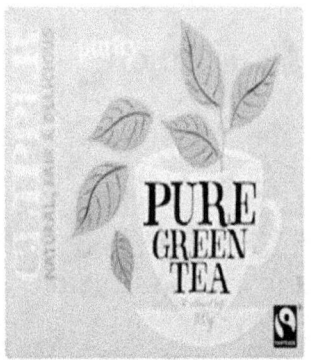

From, powerful antioxidants and nutrients to improved brain function, fat loss, and lowering the risk of cancer.

Green tea contains polyphenols like flavonoids and catechin's, which function as powerful antioxidants.

They help mop-up free radicals, which are known to play a role in the aging process.

Free radicals are produced every time we breathe oxygen, and roam around the body obliterating cells.

Green tea acts like a stimulant, having a beneficial effect on the memory, including improved moods, vigilance, reaction times, and anti-anxiety effects.

There are some studies that suggest that green tea may protect us from old age related diseases like Alzheimer's and Parkinson's?

There have been many studies demonstrating green teas abilities to burn off body fat and increase energy levels.

Green tea has been shown to heighten the metabolic rate and boost fat burning in the short term, because green tea is packed full of very powerful antioxidants.

There is a case, and some research, that supports the notion that green tea may very well be an excellent agent for reducing and protecting us against the risk of cancers.

Cancers like; breast cancer, prostate, and colorectal cancer.

There have been many studies showing the beneficial properties of taking green tea.

But one of the most interesting studies carried out, indicates that green tea may have some very powerful anti-bacteria properties.

These properties may have the ability to kill off germs, and restrain viruses like the influenza virus, and potentially lowering your risk of infections... it's a great way to help cure bad breath too.

Some real exciting news came from a review carried out on 7 different studies, involving a total of 286,701 individuals, which showed that drinking green tea lowered the risk of becoming diabetic by around **18%**.

But did you know that research has also shown that green tea may also protect us from **'STROKES'**?

For more information or to purchase your own supply, please copy this link into your browser...

http://mybooksupply.com/wp/green-tea

MAGNESIUM

Release Energy and Boost HGH

Athletes use magnesium to help increase energy output and improve their endurance.

Magnesium is required for the proper growth and maintenance of bones, proper function of nerves, and muscles.

Magnesium helps to neutralize stomach acid and works as a laxative to move stools through the intestine, helping the detoxification of the body.

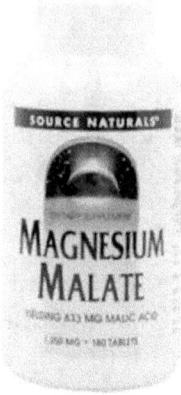

Magnesium is also involved in the production of enzymes (Enzymes are protein molecules that stimulate every chemical reaction in the body); it also assists with thousands of others too. Increases Insulin-like Growth Factors (IGF-1) levels, prevents muscle cramps, reduces lactic acid build-up, migraines, fatigue, increases bone strength, loss of appetite, or high blood pressure.

Magnesium is an essential mineral to maintaining a healthy body and lifestyle.

For more information or to purchase your own supply, please copy this link into your browser...

http://mybooksupply.com/wp/magnesium

A Quick Summery so Far

Love them, hate them, supplements have been around for a long time now and look set to go for some time to come. Supplements have a place in the diet routines of these who have embarked upon any health or weight training program.

For those of you who wish to lose pounds from your bodies and not your pockets, I hope you are able to use the above Information to good effect.

It's not necessary to take all the above supplements, only these you believe will help you in your fight to win your goals.

But do remember how important it is to read the labels on the bottles of these fat-burning, or any supplements, you may be thinking of buying.

You now have a better understanding of what a good or bad supplement has to offer you before you buy it, you are now better able to decipher the difference between an ineffective supplement and one that will yield results.

But we are not quite finished just yet, below is an index of the roll vitamins have to play in your quest for perfection, and their importance for a healthy body and mind.

Let's jump right into this fascinating world of 'Vitamins'!

VITAMINS

Getting The Right Amount Of Vitamins

Normally, and as a rule of thumb, if you are eating a healthy, balanced meal each and every day, you will be getting all of the necessary vitamins and minerals your body needs to function properly.

That is unless you exercise, *'Why'*, because training and taking supplements, will deplete your vitamin and mineral levels faster than you can replace them through your meals.

And even though we all have different dietary needs, we all need vitamins in order to live healthy lives and prevent diseases.
You need a certain amount of vitamins to keep your body healthy, and there are a lot of different vitamins out there to choose from.

But which ones should you be taking to help maintain balance.

Vitamins are very important to the health of your body, and they come under different classifications, A, B, C, and E, each one serving a different unique function.

Some are water soluble and others are oil soluble, but don't let all this worry you, because we are going to take a closer look at each one in turn, to evaluate their functions and their importance to you, the trainee.

Vitamin A

You can find vitamin A in natural foods such as oranges and yellow fruits, including vegetables, such as spinach, and some fats too.

Vitamin A is required to maintain healthy skin and keep your eyesight sharp.

Protein combines with vitamin A to make it stronger, and helps it move through your body.

This is important, because when you train, even if only doing low level exercise, you will create micro tears in muscle and surrounding soft tissue, and protein is required to repair these tears.

Deficiency in vitamin A can lead to skin problems, increased infections, and even night blindness as well.

Vitamin B

There are eight B vitamins in all, B1, B2, B3, B5, B6, B7, B9, B12, are very often referred to as **'Vitamin B complex'**. They play a very important role in keeping our bodies running at tip, top condition.

They help convert our food into fuel, keeping us energized throughout the day.

They all work together, in sequence, but doing their own specific thing.

Their rolls can be anything from promoting healthy skin, hair, nails, creating hormones to preventing memory loss.

For example:

B1 (Thiamine)

Vitamin B1 is important, because it helps to protect our immune system, so it's sometimes referred to as an Anti-stress hormone.

B1 also helps to breakdown simple carbs; these are carbohydrates that absorb quickly into the blood providing a boost of energy when needed. B1 is also responsible for building new cells.

Foods that are high sources of B1: peanuts, beans, spinach, kale, blackstrap molasses and wheat germ.

B2 (Riboflavin)

Vitamin B2 acts as an antitoxin and is very good at fighting free radicals, particles created when you burn oxygen as fuel.

They then go on to damage cells throughout the body, therefore, may help to prevent heart disease and the early signs of ageing.

Vitamin B2 is also important in the production of red blood cells, which transport oxygen throughout the body.

There are some studies that may indicate that B2 can help relieve migraines.

Foods that contain vitamin B2: soya beans, spinach, Brussels sprouts, wild rice, milk, almonds, yoghurt, and eggs.

B3 (Niacin)

One of vitamins B3 primary functions is to boost the cholesterol HDL levels. This is important, because the higher a person's HDL levels, the less bad cholesterol there will be in their blood system.

Vitamin B3 has also been used to treat acne.

Foods that are high sources of B3: eggs, beans, yeast, red meat, milk, and green vegetable.

B5 (Pantothenic Acid)

Vitamin B5 primary function is the production of sex and

stress related hormones, which include testosterone.

Research has also shown that B5 helps to promote healthy skin by reducing the signs of ageing, redness and skin spots.

For example, vitamin B5 helps to breakdown fats and carbohydrates for energy.

Foods that are high sources of B5: meet, eggs, avocados, yoghurt.

B6 (Pyridoxine)

Vitamin B6 helps to regulate the levels of the amino acid Homocysteine, which is associated with heart disease.

It also plays a primary role in producing the stress hormones serotonin, melatonin and norepinephrine.

These are important hormones as they play an important role in sleep patterns and mood swings.

Some research as shown that vitamin B6 directly reduces the effects of inflammation of those suffering from rheumatoid arthritis.

Foods containing high sources of B6: cheese, salmon, chicken, turkey, brown rice, lentils, sunflower seeds, tuna, and carrots.

B7 (Biotin)

Vitamin B7 is also known as the 'Beauty vitamin', because of its association with healthy skin, hair, and nails.

There is some research that indicates that vitamin B7 may

help to reduce high blood glucose levels.

Foods containing high levels of B7: barley, yeast, pork, fish, cauliflower, egg yolks, potatoes, chicken, liver, and nuts.

B9 (Folate)

Vitamin B9, or folic acid, is important for women who are pregnant; because B9 helps cells divide properly without developing defects.

Studies have shown that Vitamin B9 is involved in helping to prevent memory loss and keep depression at bay.

It's used extensively in fortified foods like cereals and breads.

Foods containing high levels of B9: salmon, root vegetables, milk, beans, asparagus, dark greens, and wheat.

B12 (Cobalamin)

Vitamin B12 is a very important vitamin as Cobalamin works in conjunction with vitamin B9 and helps to produce red blood cells.

It also helps iron in the blood to do its job, creating oxygen carrying protein, hemogloblin.

It's also important for maintaining the nervous systems, which sends messages to and from the brain to tell us that things are hot, painful, itchy, moving, and so forth.

Although, vitamin B12 can be stored in the body, in some cases, it's not used correctly; therefore, it's important to get a daily supply of B12 as our bodies cannot function properly if levels get depleted.

Foods containing high levels of B7: beef and pork, eggs, fish, dairy products, shellfish, and milk.

Vitamin C

Vitamin C, or L-ascorbic acid, is basically an antioxidant; it helps to protect our bodies from free radicals that damage cells in our bodies.

This property may specifically be linked to reducing the signs of aging.

Vitamin C has also been linked to a cure for the common cold.

The benefits of taking vitamin C are; it helps to protect against immune system deficiencies, cardiovascular disease, eye disease, and wrinkling skin.

Because vitamin C is water soluble, large amounts of it gets expelled through the urine and therefore, it needs to be taken on a daily basis.

Research has also shown that Vitamin C may help to improve the healing process of cuts and broken bones, to burns, and recovery from surgical wounds.

VITAMIN C taken orally can help wounds to heal faster and *BETTER*.

Foods containing high levels of Vitamin C are: green peppers, citrus fruits, strawberries, green vegetables, fish, potatoes, broccoli, milk, and tomatoes.

Vitamin D

Vitamin D is an extremely important vitamin the body requires to carry out some very major functions throughout the body, which you are about to discover.

There are two main forms of vitamin D, they are D2 and D3.

Some of these are produced when you are exposed to sunlight, which means that sunlight might be an important part of your vitamin D intake.

In general Vitamin D helps to control the calcium and the phosphorus levels in your blood.

This is important, because the Vitamin D essentially supports the way that the calcium and phosphorus are absorbed from the food you eat, into your intestines.

It also plays an important role in helping the calcium be reabsorbed in your kidneys.

Another important role that Vitamin D plays in your body is the promotion of your bone formation, and the mineralization of the skeletal system.

It also plays a big role in promoting the immune system and a big role in anti-tumour activity.

The most important Vitamin D your body requires is, D2 and D3.

D2 is not produced by the body, but comes from fungus and plant sources. Vitamin D3 is created from animal sources, and it can be made in your skin when the right particles in your skin react with the ultraviolet light that comes from sun light.

Getting the right amounts of Vitamin D can be tricky, but it is a very important vitamin you require. It might be hard for you to get just the right amount of Vitamin D, but this is where supplements can come in handy.

Foods containing high levels of Vitamin C: salmon, cod liver oil, oily fish, mushrooms, fortified cereals, Tofu, caviar, dairy products, pork, eggs, yoghurt, and sunlight.

Vitamin E

Vitamin E is a fat-soluble vitamin, which means it can be stored in the body for later use, it's important to know that Vitamin E is made in the body,

Therefore, we do not have to eat foods rich in vitamin E every single day.

Vitamin E is another antioxidant. Also vitamin E plays a supportive role helping the body use vitamin K, which helps your blood clot.

Vitamin E helps boost the immune system, helping the body to fight off bacteria's and infections.

In addition, cells use vitamin E to communicate with one another and to carry out many essential operations.

Foods especially rich in vitamin E include: wheat germ, corn, asparagus, vegetable oils, olives, margarine, nuts, and leafy green vegetables, like spinach.

I sincerely hope you enjoyed reading this book and acquired some value from it, and will continual to use this book for further reference to supplements and vitamins.

Judge J

Grab Your FREE Copy of
'Healthy Recipes Healthy Life's'

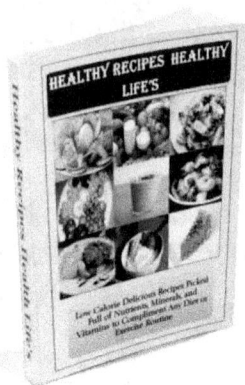

A <u>FREE</u> Health Recipe Book

It Will Make Your Mouth Water
& Keep You Healthy Too

Your **'FREE'** gift... **'Healthy Recipes Healthy Life's'** this a free **RECIPE** book packed full of tasty, delicious, filling healthy food recipes, and facts, to help you manage your weight better, after all... **'We Are What We Eat'.**

Each recipe contains full calorie count, fat, sodium, cholesterol, fibre, sugar, protein values, for your guidance. And that's not all; find out **'What'** the health benefits of herbals and spices used in these recipes.

Download your **FREE** book; copy this link into your browser...

http://eepurl.com/ct1GMH

Further reading...

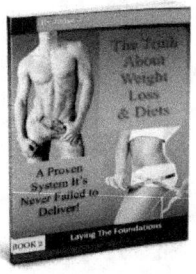

Truth About Weight Loss & Diets examines and addresses the fundamentals of diets. Going straight onto a diet is asking to fail. It's important to understand the physical and mental restraints a diet will place upon your body and 'How' to deal with them.

Examining everything from foods to eat and foods you shouldn't, to weight lose & bodybuilding myths, how much food you need to eat, essential fatty acids, proteins & carbohydrates, why dieting doesn't work, do you really lose weight drinking water, green tea, supplementation, and so much more.

For more information copy this link into your browser... http://mybooksupply.com/wp/truth-about-weight-loss

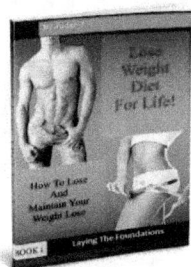

Lose Weight Diet For Life. When thinking for going on a diet, it's very important to plan your way ahead. Dieting is by its very nature very stressful on your body and mind and is a minefield of traps that will have you quitting your diet before you have hardly begun.

If you have found yourself yo-yoing, in and out of a diet, or just thinking about starting one, you will need to build a strong foundation, one which will support your efforts, keeping you on the straight and narrow throughout your weight loss campaign. Don't keep falling into the same old traps, you know they don't work. Give yourself a fighting chance...

For more information copy this link into your browser... http://mybooksupply.com/wp/diet-for-life

If you enjoyed reading my work, please feel free to check out my other book titles, visit my Website at:

http://mybooksupply.com (a work in progress)

You can also follow me on –

'Twitter': @hotwealth
'LinkedIn': http://uk.linkedin.com/in/judgej
'Facebook': https://www.facebook.com/pages/Lose-weight-manage-weight/343091449182861

'Why' Not Get Your '<u>Free</u>' Health App – Now

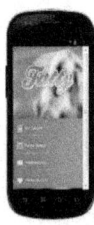
Keep yourself up-to-date with our Free *Health App*... 'Your Health Coach' Copy the <u>link below</u> visit the 'Google Play Store' - for your 'Free Health App' download...

https://play.google.com/store/apps/details?id=com.squeeze mobi.yourhealthcoach

We wish you the best of luck in building your own weight management system!

And I look forward to helping you explore, expand, and develop your weight management strategies in my next book... *My personal wishes in all your endeavours!*

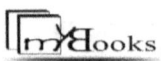

www.ingramcontent.com/pod-product-compliance
Lightning Source LLC
Chambersburg PA
CBHW071254280526
45788CB00004B/1719